BRIDGE OF SKILLS

By
Linda Chatelain

BRIDGE OF SKILLS
Copyright © 2013 by Linda Chatelain

ISBN 978-1-938669-00-2

Dedicated to:

Elaine and Mike Blymiller for their love and support in encouraging me to take a new look at my life. I want to thank Elaine for her continuing support as I continually learn to live life in new ways. I thank her for her support in encouraging me to use and share my talents in ways that will inspire and encourage others.

Darren Leighton who was my buddy during a training. Darren has remained a cherished friend and an example to me of continually looking for someone to share happiness with. Many of the principles I live by today, I learned while he held my hand in friendship and belief.

TABLE OF CONTENTS

LOOK IN THE MIRROR OFTEN

RESPONSIBLE CHOICES

TAKE RESPONSIBILITY

THERE IS A CHOICE

ALLOW OTHERS TO HAVE PROBLEMS

STAND BACK AND STEP AWAY

LET GO AND LET...

MANAGE THE FEELING

STOP DROP AND ROLL

LIVE THROUGH THE FEELING

FORGIVE

SOMETHING FOR YOU

TREAT YOURSELF

STOP AND BE A CHILD

LAUGH AT LIFE

KEEP THE SCALES IN BALANCE

FILL THE TANKS OFTEN

SERVE SOMEONE ELSE

BE GRATEFUL

WRITE IT DOWN

IT IS PERFECT

BUILD A BRIDGE FOR OTHERS

INTRODUCTION

Recently I shared with someone I thought I trusted an idea I had to share some of my experiences in life with others who might be looking for encouragement. His reaction was to ask me why I thought someone would even care about what I had to say. He reminded me that as far as he was concerned, I didn't have impressive credentials to show or a list of degrees to display. I told him that evening that I felt I had a lot to share simply because I had gone through many trials and experiences and in-spite of everything I had gone through I was still standing and could possibly give some encouragement to others that they can make it through whatever the pressures they are presently feeling.

I went home that evening with this gentleman's question still on my mind. Why did I think I had something to share that might help lift another person's heart or assist them in finding even a small amount of peace in their life? The answer came again, simply and quietly, into my heart. I could reach out and offer hope because I had been in a similar situation and know there is hope. I was able to find hope when it was difficult to believe and so I can offer that same hope to someone else still searching. I can identify with many who are co-dependent to a loved one caught in a destructive cycle. I can identify with the women who is struggling with the feelings and decisions of being abused or watching your children be abused. I can identify with the single mother who is starting over and doesn't know where or who to turn to. I can understand the feelings of a mother coping with a child with physical, emotional or learning disabilities because I have walked their path before them. I know what many of these people are going through, particularly as a woman. I may not be an expert, but I have the power to teach and inspire others because I know what works for me. I know that you can make it through one more day, whether you want to or not, and still remain standing as a survivor.

I have heard life referred to as a roller-coaster ride. With all the ups and downs, turns and twists it is an appropriate way of describing the feeling that there is always one more adventure, one more thrill waiting to surprise us for as long as the ride goes on. Life is also like an ongoing baseball game. You are thrown curves and challenges every inning. Sometimes the ball of life passes you by, sometimes we swing and strike out but most of the time if we focus ourselves and stay steady we can hit that ball into the outfield or even make a homerun. Life has also been described as a journey through valleys of despair and mountains of joy. It is a journey where the highways of life we choose at the forks of life can lead almost anywhere, have potholes to get stuck in and straight-a-ways for racing ahead on.

However we describe life, there is one truth in common. Life is unpredictable. We need to have skills that will help us to climb, slow our falls, dig our way out of the pits and just keep moving onward and forward on our individual paths.

One of my favorite songs as a child was the song "The Bridge Builder." I loved the song because it showed the caring we should have one for another. I also loved it because I was close to my grandfather and this song reminded me of him. Following is a copy of the poem I saved.

THE BRIDGE BUILDER

An old man, going a lone highway,

Came at evening time, cold and gray

To a chasm, vast and deep and wide,

Through which was flowing a sullen tide.

The old man crossed in the twilight dim;

The sullen stream had no fears for him;

But he turned when safe on the other side

And built a bridge to span the tide.

"Old man," said a fellow pilgrim near,

"You are wasting your strength with building here;

Your journey will end with the closing day;

You never again must pass this way;

You have crossed the ravine, deep and dark and wide.

Why build you the bridge at the eventide?"

The builder lifted his old gray head:
"Good friend in the path I have come," he said,
"There followeth after me today
A youth whose feet must pass this way.
This chasm that was as naught to me
To that fair-haired youth may a pit-fall be,
He, too, must cross in the twilight dim;
Good friend, I'm building this bridge for him."
By Will Allen Dromgoole

I have thought about the message of this song many times the past few weeks as I have pondered my friend's question of who would benefit from my writing. The words that kept coming to my mind were the last four lines. In this song the builder is thinking of someone who will go in the path he has followed. He builds a bridge to help the youth to get across the chasm with ease. Just as when I was a child, these thoughts touched my heart deeply. Rereading this song strengthened my desire to share my experiences and the lessons I have learned with others. I am so grateful to the teachers of my life, those who helped me know the way over and around the rocks. The best way I know to thank them is to pass their gifts on. It is my turn to be a guide to others who are now crossing the same paths or may need a bridge of faith or skill to get them over the sullen waters and the ravine so vast, deep and wide.

There is an ancient saying that when a dove flaps its wings in china the wind currents shift for thousands of miles across mountains and seas. Everything we do has a ripple effect. Many times I have been shown the example of the ripple effect. I have watched as you drop a pebble into a still lake how the effect ripples outward and expands in ever increasing waves. The same holds true as we touch another life. We may never know the difference that we made to someone else we never know simply because we touched the surface of one life with love. If I can touch even one heart through the words I write I will be successful in sending love to ripple on. If even one person reading these thoughts is lifted to search for a better path or a new way of being then what I have gone through and what I share can be the beginning of a new ripple of joy. If even one person reaches a little higher, looks a little deeper within or takes one more step they didn't think they could take, then a ripple of strength and belief will extend in a boundless wave.

In her album, <u>Timeless, Live in Concert,</u> Barbara Streisand sings a song that is an excellent reminder to us all that we are not alone and the positive energy and love that would result if all reached out to one another.

AT THE SAME TIME

Think of all the homeless living in the world at the same time.

Think of all the faces and the stories they could tell at the same time.

Think of all the eyes looking out into this world,

Trying to make sense of what they see.

Think of all the ways you have of seeing.

Think of all the ways there are of being.

Think of all the children being born into this world at the same time.

Feel your love surround them as they fill the need to grow at the same time.

Just think of all the hands that will be reaching for a dream,

Think of all the dreams that could come true.

Yes, if the hands we're reaching with would come together joining me and you.

When it comes to thinking of tomorrow,

We must protect our fragile destiny.

In this precious life there's no time to follow

The time has come to be a family.

Think of all the love pouring from our hearts at the same time.

Yes, Think of all that love that could shine around the world at the same time.

Just think what we've been given and just think what we could
lose,
All of life is in our trembling hands,
It's time to overcome our fears and join to build the world that
loves and understands
It helps to think of all the hearts beating in the world,
And hopes in all the hearts beating in the world
There's a healing music in our hearts swelling in this world at
the same time.
At the same time.

By A. H. Calloway

LIVE ONE DAY AT A TIME

If I could share only one idea with you about life, it would be to live one day at a time. It is the secret to coping and working your way through almost any crisis. This idea and life element is consistent and has never failed to work for me, no matter what is happening in my life.

Today is here. Yesterday is gone. Tomorrow is just a dream of the future. You have today, right now, this moment. You may or may not be able to recreate a moment from the past. You may or may not be able to make a difference tomorrow. What you can do is make this moment count.

Yesterday was an important day in your life. All the yesterdays of your life have brought you to today, one day at a time. Some days have been good, some not so good, but all have been. You learned. You grew. You changed. You hurt, loved, cried and laughed. You experienced whatever life made available for you to be a part of. You simply lived, one yesterday at a time, until you reached today. You have the hope and proof that if you could live through yesterday you can live through today. As the sun rises in the morning you will be able to stand, look back and say, I lived through yesterday so I can live through today.

Tomorrow is an illusion. It is beyond your present grasp. You can plan for it. You can wish for it. You can offer promises of what is to come. You can work today to make something that may happen tomorrow. You can hope that tomorrow will be different. You can perform all kinds of exercises or activities to prepare for tomorrow. What you cannot do is live tomorrow. When the morning sun of tomorrow rises you find you are at the beginning of a new today. Tomorrow is still a day away. You have to live in today.

So you live one day a time. You can look back at yesterday for the lessons, if you want to. You can even dream about tomorrow if you desire. The key though, is to live one day. Just live through today. One day at a time you choose how you will use your time, talents, resources and energy. One day at a time choose how you act, how you react to a feeling or situation. One day at a time you can make it past yesterday and to tomorrow.

Life is a series of days. You cannot live more than once day at a time. You cannot live in yesterday, today and tomorrow at the same time. So simply live one day at a time. Make it through whatever life hands you today. Then do it again tomorrow. Use the wisdom and knowledge, the skills, the strength you gain today to make it through one more day when it arrives. For one day let yourself believe that the next day can and will be different. For one day live in the moment of now. For one day pause and let sunshine warm your soul. For one day let life happen as it will. For one day decide to stop your self-defeating habits and thoughts. For one day reach out to someone else. For one day let go of stress and worry. For one day forgive yourself. For one day stand firm in your beliefs. What ever it is you want, do it for just one day. Yesterday is gone and tomorrow will come on its own. So for just today, live one day. .

I live my own life one day at a time. I have not found any other way to live. With all the stress I feel each day, the decisions I feel I need to make and the responsibilities I am expected to fulfill, I choose to live just one day at a time. I know that I may have made mistakes in a choice I made yesterday or the day before but I can't go back and change them. I have already created the results so today I must decide what to do. Some days I choose not to do anything. For today I might not call a daughter to discuss visitation issues because I choose today to avoid the stress of dealing with the usual anger that ensues. I have to choose my priorities. For today is it more important to send out resumes and look for work, or more important to be available to meet with a school teacher? Sometimes it is a choice of not choosing at all, of waiting to see how things will work out before I step in or make a choice. For today I can let my daughter find her own way of handling disturbing medical news without offering any solutions or becoming co-dependent. For one day I can let myself have fun with the children and allow work to wait for tomorrow without guilt. For one day I can devote myself to work all day and know that tomorrow there will be time to relax without feeling I am cheating myself or my family. For one day I can stand firm in enforcing visitation issues. For one day I can do my best to improve, to let go of a bad habit or to attempt something new. By taking one day at a time I know I don't have to last any longer than the present 16 hours of the day I am not sleeping. It doesn't really matter what the day brings I can handle anything for one day and so can you.

ONLY YOU ARE YOU

BE WHO YOU ARE

You are a unique individual unlike anyone else anywhere else in this world. You may share some traits with someone else, but no one is exactly you. No one has the same features, personalities, talents, abilities, skills, mind or thoughts as you do. You are not anyone else but yourself.

It is okay to simply be you. You cannot be anyone else beside who you are, so come to peace with yourself. You cannot be someone else because they are already themselves, so stop trying to be the perfect neighbor you think you see next door. You cannot be exactly who someone else thinks you should be because you may not get to have all the advantages they expect you to have to get there. Life does not always happen according to someone else's expectations. It is okay to be you living your life. It is okay to be who you are right now. Give yourself permission to accept yourself as you are right now. It is okay to have flaws, faults and imperfections. That is part of what makes you different than anyone else. It is okay to be different.

Accepting and being who you are is the beginning of allowing change. Accepting and being who you are at this moment is your basis for comparison as you grow and learn. If I accept that I presently weigh 165 pounds. wear a size 16 and feel like that is perfect for me right now, I appreciate more when I am able to lose a small five pounds. To me five pounds I have not lost in several years is a real accomplishment I can be proud of. An alcoholic has to admit who they are and love himself as an alcoholic, before he can increase his love enough to seek intervention. No improvement program will work until you are able to accept and love who you are at the start. You cannot become someone better unless you are being someone already.

Be who you are first, and then seek for improvement. If you have a lot of pent up anger then be angry. After you feel the anger you can then look for ways to manage the anger in appropriate ways. If you are sad, then be sad while looking for ways to find happiness. If you do not feel you can look like a magazine model then be a real-life model. Be who you are now, wearing what you enjoy, with a smile. You may find that you don't have to make any change to be the perfect model for your size and shape. If you are happy and enjoy being with your family more than cleaning the house all day, then be someone who is happy when she is with her family. If you find you are someone who enjoys reading, then be a reader. If you are a perfectionist, then be as perfect as you can as you learn to accept that we cannot all be perfect all the time. Start from where you are, be who you are and then love who you are.

BE UNIQUE

Since there is only one you in this world, it makes perfect sense to be unique. Find something about yourself that you can develop and showcase in an easy manner. Everyone has some trait that someone else admires or wishes they had. Talk with friends and family to see what they admire about you. Build on your special talents, traits, and abilities. The more unique you feel the more love you will find you have for yourself. The more special you feel you are, the more self-confidence you will find bubbling forth.

Ask yourself what you can make uniquely yours. What do you feel others first notice about you? Make that trait a signature item that works for you. Perhaps your hair is long and silky. Find a style of your own that shows off your tresses. If you have a flair for talking with people, become known as the person who will be the first one to greet a new employee, a new member of the club or a stranger at a party. Create your own fashionable clothing style that brings out your most attractive traits. If you have a sense of humor, be unique in putting others at ease in stressful situations. Use your individualism to inspire others. Your individuality may be the inspiration to another person to try something new, something they have been thinking about doing or something they have always wanted to be. You never know who you may touch.

FIND THE STRENGTH WITHIN

You might have to dig through a pile of fears, worry and false beliefs, but underneath it all is your own personal gift to yourself. Deep within you is the strength to hold on to life, to take one more step and endure one minute more. Within you is a strength you may have only tapped the surface of. It may be buried deep, so deep you are barely aware of it as you try to hang on emotionally or physically from day to day. It may be just below the surface of frustration or sorrow but it is within waiting for you to search it out.

The strength within you may be different than someone else's. I may have the strength to hold my temper and keep my feelings in check during stressful situations. You may have the strength to be able to speak your mind and heart in the same situations. Whatever your strength, it is right for you. I may have the strength to listen to an angry child without feeling I am a failure while you may have the strength to face an angry child and powerfully confront the issues head-on. You may have the strength to move mountains while I may have the strength to tunnel a way through. Our strengths may be different for we are each different. So accept the strengths you are aware of.

Find the strength you need by seeking within. You always have the strength you need but sometimes you may not look deep enough or even look for it at all. If you need the strength to leave an abusive relationship you will find it if you look. If you need the strength to stand alone and walk forward you will find it within. Within is where you will find the strength to solve one more problem or face one more crisis with courage and hope. If you look within you will find the strength to lift not only yourself but also those you love from the depths of sorrow or suffering. Whatever the strength you need to find, it will be there if make the effort to look for it. Receive the gift you have been saving for that rainy day that just arrived.

NEVER GIVE UP ON YOURSELF

You are worth loving and making a difference. When others give up on you have faith in yourself you can make a difference. No one is you but you. No one can motivate you better than yourself. You are the only one that knows what is in your heart, your reason for going on from day to day or how you accomplish what you do. When it seems like no one thinks you can, don't give up on yourself.

When it seems that everyone else has given up on you, have faith in yourself that you can reach your goals. Don't give up on a dream of personal change just because someone else does not believe you are capable of making the goal. Show them you were right all along. When it seems that there are little that believe that you are trying your best don't give up on yourself to keep giving everything you have to give. Only you know what your best is and your best will always influence and count to those who will be influential in your life.

No one knows you better than yourself. You are the one that knows if you are trying your best. Don't give up on yourself when you know that what you are working for is worthwhile. Others can withdraw their support or encouragement but only you can truly give up on yourself. Others can not see what is in your heart and mind. Find your personal reasons and what motivates you. As long as you have any reason for what you are doing, do not give up. Never give up on your own potential to use your strengths, talents, abilities and knowledge. You are the only person with your knowledge and power. No one can take them away from you. So don't give up on you. Give yourself one more push, one more cheer and go for the win.

TRUST YOURSELF ONCE IN A WHILE

You have heard someone plead to "trust me." How many times have you given your trust to other people? You often trust the judgment, opinions or direction of others. Sometimes all someone needs to receive your trust is the approval of another person you already trust. If they give you permission you often will trust without question. All too often though, you do not trust your own judgments, opinions or direction. You somehow feel that your ideas or feelings are less important or worthy of faith than someone else with more power, influence or knowledge.

Don't always rely on the thoughts, opinions or direction of others. Trust yourself once in a while to make the right decision for you. Others may be pushing you to change this way or that. Let them have their opinions. Realize that no two people are the same and no two people think or feel the same. Everyone is in unique circumstances with elements that influence the outcome differently even in similar situations. The answer cannot always be the same for everyone. Once in a while trust the fact that only you know what your feelings are. Only you know what you want or need at any given time. Only you know what you can handle at the time along with everything else life is offering you so trust your own opinions and thoughts. Many a man has been scammed because he invested in a plan someone else trusted even when his own mind was screaming out this opportunity was not all it appeared to be.

Trust yourself to follow your own beliefs, your own path or your own way of being you. No one else is you or can be you 100 percent of the time. As you learn to trust your own feelings you will find that your intuition becomes stronger and more frequent. The more you trust your feelings the more you know you can depend on your own truths. So take the first step. Trust yourself as much as you trust others, at least once in a while.

TAKE A STEP

ONE STEP AT A TIME

Take life one step at a time. Solve a problem one step at a time. A baby does not come into this world walking. A baby learns one step at a time. Watch the progress of a baby through his first year as he goes from lying still to rolling over to sitting up to pulling himself up to inching along holding on to someone or something strong, to risking one step and then another until he finally can take one step after another and keep on moving and then take one step after another faster and faster until he is running. Life is no different. We all go through stages of growth in order to become who or what we are. Just take one stage or one step at a time.

Each of us has our own paths to walk. My path may seem rocky and steep. Your path may seem downhill and smooth. My path may have twists and turns at every corner while yours may seem to reach on endlessly before you. As different as our paths may be we all must traverse them in the same way. You can only move forward or backward by taking a step. Sometimes as one problem follows another in a series of events you feel like you are taking one step back. It may even feel like many. Sometimes one step back is just putting your feet together to regain balance so you can move with more surety or strength. .

Recognize you have come a long way and may have a way to go yet but you are taking the next step and others will come when you are ready and willing. You begin to dance through life but if you look down at our feet you realize even in dancing you are taking only one step at a time followed by more steps.

It only takes one small step to begin a journey. Until you take that first step you are going nowhere. When you look at where you want to be you often count how many steps it will take, become discouraged and never begin the journey. Taking the first step to recovery from an addiction is often the hardest one to take. The first step may often be the one that takes the greatest courage. Once taken the next steps are easy to make one at a time. Raising yourself up means not only taking one step at a time but requires you step higher each time. Whether climbing a flight of stairs or a ladder, it still takes one step and then another to get to the top.

Recognize with each step that you have come a long way. You may have a long way to go but each step take you further. It doesn't matter whether the steps are big or small as long as they are taken. It doesn't matter if you stop to rest between the steps, as long as you keep on stepping. If you aren't sure what the next step is ahead, take one anyway. When your foot hits the ground you will be in a new place and once step ahead of where you thought you could be.

TAKE ONE MORE STEP

When you feel like you just can't go on any longer take one more step. When you feel you can't go any further then take just one more step. Give yourself one more chance. Give yourself one more burst of love. Like the marathon runner at the end of the race, one more step can get you across the finish line. When you take that one more step give yourself credit and celebrate.

Taking one more step means you have not given up. Taking one more step is proof positive you can give more than you thought. Taking one more step shows you are willing to give your all and a little more when needed. Taking one more step is a reminder if you can do something once, you can do it again. Take one more step and find out the power it gives you in overcoming the trials of life.

IT DOESN'T HAVE TO LOOK A CERTAIN WAY

This is one of the greatest lessons I learned myself a few years ago. I use this principle when I am stuck in whatever is going on in my life. I use it to get myself past what others think they are seeing that may not be so. I use this principle when I am stuck in performing the way I think I am supposed to. I use this principle when someone who thinks they know what the end looks like tells me what I should be doing or how I should be doing it. Any time I am stuck in have to, should, supposed to or must, I remind myself "It doesn't have to look a certain way."

Just because someone else sees the box as a closed square, you do not have to see it the same way. You can see the flaps that open and close the box. You can look to see the color or a pattern they aren't seeing or overlooked. Just because you want it to look brown doesn't mean it has to be brown. A white box carries as much trash to the curb as a brown one does. You can fill it just as full. It is just the same weight, it just looks different. So it is with life. Just because you think something has to look a certain way doesn't mean it does or must. .

I learned this principle while attending some personal trainings a few years ago. Learning this principle changed my life. Knowing the outcome and circumstances do no have to look a certain way allowed me to start accepting the results as they came without looking for something different. I stopped looking for what I thought should be happening and started accepting what was happening with a calm mind. I stopped worrying so much about what other people thought or wanted. I started trusting that even if what I thought was different than expected I was okay and the idea was worthwhile. Learning this principle allowed me to accept and love what I already had and stop defeating myself by comparing myself to others, always wishing my circumstances were different. Releasing the need to have things a certain way brought a peace that I was worthwhile and was doing what was perfect for me to be doing, even if it was not what someone else would do I the same circumstances.

Make this principle a part of your life. See what freedom it allows you in making choices that are not exact matches to how someone else would live your life. When I was working with some home aides a few months ago, one of our problem areas was my daughter's room. To them clean and neat meant her dresser would be clear and orderly. They envisioned everything behind a closet door. I knew their vision would not work for this daughter. Instead of building shelves in the closet for her to store things on where she needed to get up from bed and walk across the room to get anything or put anything away, I created a storage center for her on the dresser. The bins and drawers are just steps from her bedside, sorted into small groups so she can easily get to the items without removing a lot of other items which probably would not get put away immediately. The end result was not what the aides originally had in mind, but when it was complete they agreed it worked well and still looked neat.

Remember it doesn't have to look a certain way. See for yourself the freedom this phrase will give you in your life. Use this phrase whenever you are stressed or worried about how something is supposed to be, look or come about. You will find the choices you can make are limitless when you are not bound to only a few acceptable results. When all results are acceptable, if they work for you and others, then new worlds of opportunities open up.

THERE IS MORE THAN ONE WAY

There is no right or wrong way to do something or reach a goal. There are many different ways. Some ways may work for you, others may not. Even if you do not do something a certain way, that way is still an option for someone else or for another time when it may work better.

During a training I took a few years ago I participated in an exercise where 70 people had to cross a room. No two people could cross in the same one way. If you crossed in a way someone else did, such as walking, you had to change something about it. (If the other person swung his arms while walking then you could cross your arms and walk across) I learned there were at least 70 ways, 70 choices that could be made in order to get to the other side, to end up at the same place with everyone else. The lesson was simple, there is more than one way to get where you want to go. If one way is not working or someone has already tried that way, think again. Learn from someone else, make a simple difference, then get to the destination your own way. There are as many ways of doing something or getting somewhere as there are people.

Find as many ways as you can of getting something done. Be open to something different happening. Try something no one else has tried before. You can get a clean floor whether you use a straw broom, a bristle broom, a duster or a vacuum. The end is the same the difference is the method. So realize you are free to do it whenever, wherever or in whatever way works for you in your circumstances.

STEP LEFT AND GO

Not all of us are athletes that can jump every hurdle, climb any wall or run the distance. When faced with an obstacle, there will be times you do not have the strength to step over it. The best way is to go around it. Maybe the only way is to go around it. So step left or step right and go around. Give yourself permission to not punish by forcing yourself to climb the wall or trudge up and over the mountain.

It might take you longer to go around the mountain than it takes someone else to go over and down the other side but you both still arrive on the other side in due time. Perhaps around is the simpler way. Do we all have to fight the rocks and crags, take the risk or find the adventure? No, it is okay to step left and simply walk around on occasion. There is still beautiful scenery to enjoy and the journeys end is the same. The only difference is the way in which we made the journey.

Step left and proceed again. It sounds like a move in a game. Some of us reach a stumbling block, someone in our pathway or a small obstacle before us. We wait for the person before us to move or take a turn before us. We don't consider if we move and proceed, perhaps we can walk and learn together. Before I learned this principle I would often stumble and fall over the blocks of life or bump my head repeatedly against the obstacle hoping for it to just go away. Now as I see the obstacles or stumbling blocks I can sometimes step left and pass them by. When driving on a two lane highway you give yourself permission to pass an obstacle in the road or a slower vehicle by simply switching lanes and going forward. Give yourself permission to do the same in life. Step left and choose to pass by some of the obstacles and challenges you see ahead. Give yourself permission to not hit every bump in the road just because it is there. Give yourself permission to take a different route. You may even find there is a tunnel through.

LISTEN

BE STILL

Every once in a while, stop, be silent and listen. Stop and let the silence of peace, calm, serenity and stillness envelope you. Stop and just listen to the gentle sounds of nature surround you in their beauty. Listen to the wind rustling the leaves of a tree as it passes by. Listen to a drip, drip of water falling from one leaf to another after a rain shower. Listen to the quiet falling of snowflakes joining together to blanket your world in white. Stop and listen to the sounds of your home. Hear the running water of a bath waiting to cleanse. Listen to the hum of a vacuum removing debris from your life. Hear the swish, swish of a pet's tail awaiting the stroke of your loving hand. Listen to an old song and allow memories to flow through your mind. There are sounds all around to listen to if you will just stop and take a moment to listen.

Stop and let the world go on without you, around you and past you. Then open your eyes and know you are still here. You are still alive. You are still able to be a part of the world, to step right back into life. Step back on with the power of knowing life will keep going on even if you stop struggling and fighting. The merry-go-rounds of life keep on turning whether you are on them or not. It is okay to jump off for a moment, take a breath, nourish your body, mind and spirit, then climb back on again for another exciting ride. It is even okay to jump off some merry-go-rounds, such as an addictive life style or co-dependency. You do not have to ride it yourself. You can learn by watching others as they ride. The merry-go-round will keep on going for those who still enjoy the ride even without you on it.

Create a place of stillness for yourself. Find a personal escape zone. Listen to your inner knowing as it whispers to your heart of personal truth and peace. Release tension and calm the spirit. There are all kinds of ways to create or find a place of quiet for your self. I love to, in the early hours of the morning or late at night, light some candles, put on a soothing record and simply soak in a tub of warm water. I can close my eyes, feel and experience the flickering light and release all my tensions into the water or let them float away on the notes of the music. Create a mental escape you can go to whenever or wherever you need to. Think of a place that represents peace and tranquility to you personally. Envision and feel how you would want it to be if you were truly there. Draw on this vision whenever you need a moment of quiet. Have you ever taken a drive or a vacation to a memorable place in nature? Use this memory as your place of peace. Remember the sounds, the sights, the feelings you had and the people you were with that made it pleasurable. As you revisit this place in your mind you can release the present pressures and concerns to the sky, water, land or people around you.   You may already have a place of stillness and not recognize it or use it often enough. It could be a comfortable chair. I have a comfort and still zone on my bed.   As I turn the lights off each night I place the pillows behind my back, sit quietly with my hands folded across my heart and take a deep breath. In the darkness I can allow the stillness and quiet of the room to envelope me in peace. I can then lie down and go to sleep.   It doesn't matter where or what your place of stillness is. You may have many places or only one. What does matter is that you personally find a way or a place to be still; away or a place to listen for nothing or everything.

LISTEN MORE THAN YOU TALK

Someone once said "You have two ears and one mouth, use them in proportion."   I have learned it is the listening not the talking that helps me to learn more and understand more. In his book 7 Habits of Effective People, Steven Covey encourages one to seek first to understand someone and then to be understood. In order to understand you first have to listen, then make sure what you heard is what was meant, so you need to listen again. Once you are sure you understand, then you can respond and express your own thoughts.

Listen to the thoughts, feelings, desires and ideas of those around you. Listen to understand. Listen to know how someone feels, what he thinks and want he wants. Don't just listen to the words alone. Listen to the tone of the voice. Listen to the rhythm of the speech. Listen to what is not said as well as what is. Sometimes what is not said speaks louder than the words we hear. Sometimes the facial and body language are stronger than the spoken word. When you are trying to talk with someone about something you know he does not want to hear, his silence and refusal to talk tell you more about his anger than the words he retaliates with. Telling you what was said is just a bunch of nonsense tells you in words he is not open to listening to or understanding any other point of view than his own.. Averted eyes are his way of making sure you know you can talk all you want but he is not going to listen and none of what is said will make any difference in your relationship. He doesn't have to say a word. His lack of attention speaks louder than saying directly "I am not going to listen." He may talk through clenched teeth, or without moving his teeth or his lips so most of what he says is a mumble or barely able to be heard. When he talks in these ways it is not the message of the words you will hear but the tone of anger, revenge or denial. Listen not only to the messages to understand but also to the tone and the feeling of what is said. If you are not sure you understand, listen again before proceeding.

Listen to the thoughts, feelings and desires of your own heart. Listen to the feelings you have within. Listen to words you do not speak but want to or wish you could. What are these words and reactions saying to you? Listen to the words you use to describe your desires. Do you hear excitement, passion or frustration in your voice? Listen as you express thoughts and ideas. Do you speak as though you believe the ideas are good or do you keep them inside, afraid they will be rejected? What do you hear when you listen to yourself? Listen to yourself with an open mind and love in your heart. Learn about yourself from what you hear.

Listen, ponder and then listen again before you speak out in anger, in judgment or even in love. Too often individuals speak out in anger before they listen and think. Listen to the other person. Think about not only what he said but also why you feel a particular feeling? Is it what he said, how he said it or some feeling within you protected by emotion? Once you think you know why you are feeling a certain way, listen again to make sure you understood correctly before you respond. You may hear someone tell you your ideas are wrong and want to react unkindly. Listen to the inner feelings. It is not the words that your ideas are wrong you are reacting to but the feeling of being judged unfairly which triggers the feelings of anger and hurt. Recognizing this you can respond by calmly stating you understand they do not agree instead of reacting in anger and calling them names. Relationships are built on understanding and listening not on anger and reactions.

Listen to yourself, listen to another and then speak from the heart. Listen to your thoughts and feelings. Discuss them with someone you trust to treat your feelings with respect. Listen to their opinions, their thoughts, their feelings and their love. After listening then speak from your heart. Many times what you will hear yourself saying is your own thought tempered by the feelings of your trusted friend. As you speak listen to your heart. Do you hear it beating quickly in excitement or slowing in fear?

LOOK

OPEN YOUR EYES

See the beauty that is around you. Open your eyes to the beauty within you. Open your eyes and see where you are, where you can go and where others have been. See those who love you and care for you. See the world you live in. Even a blind man can open his eyes. He may not see clearly or even at all but the act itself is that of opening to see. Opening his eyes is the act of being open and ready to receive. With his eyes open he is truly more able to feel or to experience something coming his way. Open your eyes and see what is coming to you, for you and sometimes even at you.

LOOK FOR THE LESSON

Whatever you are doing, wherever you are in the experiences you are going through you are growing. You are learning. You are changing something within yourself. The change can be good or bad but there is a lesson you have the opportunity to learn. Only you can learn from the moment, from this experience in your own way. Someone else may learn for drugs give a sense of peace or calm, believing if he can't feel the pain he can go on. But someone else may be at the point of learning hiding behind the drugs is how he hides from the world and while he is hiding, others are having adventures, fun or opportunities. He learns how to come out of hiding to participate in life. Meanwhile, someone else learns hiding behind drugs is the way to lose all that is precious to him.

Look for the lessons you are learning now .Ask, "Is this what I want to learn? Is this where I want to be?" If the answer to the questions are "no," then look for the lesson you want to learn. Look for the place you want to be and learn how to get there. What lessons are you learning about the relationships you presently have? What lessons do you need to learn to have the relationships you truly want? Look for where to learn the lesson. Look for the teacher, the book or the experience that will assist you in learning a different lesson.

Look for lessons you learned in the past? All those experiences and trials you went through yesterday were for a reason. What were the lessons you learned as you went through the problems you faced and conquered? How did you survive when you didn't think you could survive any longer? What personal strengths did you learn to use that you never would have known you possessed if it had not been for the challenges you were given? These were your lessons? Did you learn them well enough you do not need to learn them again?

LOOK UP NOT DOWN

No matter where you think you are on the ladder of change, look up for the next rung. Look up at the sky and see how it goes on and on, up and up seemingly endless. Know that wherever you are, there is something higher you can reach for, climb up to or search beyond.

If you look beneath your feet you will see the ground you stand on is solid, there is nowhere to go. Now look up just a little. Where your feet meet the ground is where the sky begins. It is where you are now. The only place to go is forward and upward. From where you are you can look in any direction and move up or away. You can look up and go higher or stand still. The choice is yours. .

When you feel like you have hit bottom, look up. If you are truly at the bottom there is nowhere else to go but up. Sometimes the bottom is the only place from which you can see all the handholds needed to climb to the top. From the bottom you can see the path you need to take. Once you start the climb you will need the perspective you gained to remember and trust there is another handhold or safe ledge just a few feet above.

When you feel like you are in the depths of despair, look up. The light comes from above you not beneath you. .Remember you can only find the cloud with the silver lining if you look up.

LOOK IN THE MIRROR OFTEN

Me, myself and I looked in the mirror

Together, was the only one we saw.

Look into the mirror. See the person before you. . Do you like who you are? Are you beautiful in your own eyes? Is this person your friend? Do you trust her or hate her? When you look into the eyes, what do you see? Do you see joy, pain or someone just holding on? What can you do to let this person know you care? How do you let the person reflected know you care they are even alive? Do something for the person in the mirror. Hug her, love her, and give her encouragement and hope. Look him in the eye. Face his fears head on. Ask yourself what you think he needs and then find a way to give it to him. Find the dream for him. Simply and lovingly let him know he is not alone.

Look into the mirror. Do you see yourself as others see you? How do you present yourself? Do you dress the way you feel? Is your smile white and wide? Do you like the length, style or color of your hair? If you could change anything about the person you see in the mirror, what would it be? Ask yourself how you would like that person to look and then find a way to look the part.

RESPONSIBLE CHOICES

TAKE RESPONSIBILITY

"If not me, who?" "If not now, When?" Take responsibility for your life Take responsibility for the decisions you make. Be responsible for your actions and reactions. Be responsible for the way you feel. Take responsibility for bringing yourself to where you are now.

Don't look for someone else to blame. Take responsibility for what you are experiencing right now. Take responsibility for making a choice somewhere along the line that brought you to this point in life. No one made you do anything or took your rights away. Someone may have used tactics to induce you to choose the way you did, but you were the one that made the ultimate choice so you need to take the responsibility yourself. Take responsibility for knowing right from wrong before you made a choice. Take responsibility for errors and mistakes you have made. Don't try to find a scapegoat to carry the burden of your guilt or problems. Sometimes this is hard.

Take responsibility for your own life. Take responsibility for the reasons you to blame others. It is easier to blame others because then you don't have to feel the pain or hurt. Instead you can feel distanced from the situation by self-righteousness.

Blaming someone else is often a way of denial a problem even exists. Blaming others allows you to do the same thing again and again because it is not your fault. If you can find someone to blame you can claim you or others didn't know any better. Blaming someone else is often a tool of revenge or a means of feeling powerful. (The person feels they can hurt those they want to take the responsibility by making them feel guilty or obligated.) Blaming is often a way of demanding or asking someone else to take care of you because you cannot or are not willing to help yourself. Blaming others can be a power or control stance. (Example: "It is your fault I do not have a car. You won't buy me one so it is your fault I can't get around to get a job. Since I can't get a job it is your responsibility to pay for gas to drive me around and pay my bills for me.) It is important, in order to grow and be responsible to stop finding reasons to blame others. In blaming you mentally give your power to the other person. You deny you are a capable, powerful and knowledgeable human being. You deny you can change, grow and be happy without the assistance of others. When you stop blaming others and take responsibility for your own feelings and choices you release energy. You claim your power and release a desire to accept life as you choose it to be.

Take the responsibility for being where you are in life at this moment. Take responsibility for choices you previously made or chose not to make and the results you created. Take responsibility for the feeling or situation by knowing you called for it from others, caused it to happen or allowed it to happen in some way. Life did not just happen. It was created. Whatever situation or relationship you are involved in, take responsibility for creating the circumstances, allowing a chain of events to occur or providing a way for a a certain result to occur. Take the responsibility for allowing or asking for particular teachers to be part of your life. What lesson did you need that requires their presence?

THERE IS A CHOICE

Every moment in life offers you the opportunity to choose. You chose every day how to use each minute of each twenty-four hours we have. Sometimes the choice doesn't seem like a choice, it is just continuing with the last choice. Time just goes on. You continue doing what you were already doing, but it is a choice because at any moment you can choose to stop or to do something differently. Sometimes the act of not choosing is in fact choosing. It is the choice to do nothing, to simply flow or let things happen naturally.

How you act or react to others is a choice. Sometimes you react out of habit or seem to be on autopilot but there are still choices made in a fraction of a second to react from past experience or to act from a new perspective. You choose whether to act or react from feeling, knowledge or intuition. Whether you remain in control of your emotions or act them out is a choice. How and who you are in a relationship is a choice. You choose to be real, admitting your flaws and weaknesses, or fake, showing only either your best or your worst side. Honesty, integrity, trust, confidence and belief are all choices you get to make in relationships with others.

Everyone has the chance to make choices. You are not and should not be responsible for someone else's choices. Your son, daughter or spouse is given the opportunity to make the same kinds and the same number of choices as you are able to make. Recognize when things happen in relationships and interactions with others that both parties can and do make choices. If a relationship is not working out, realize that a choice made by the other party may be just as much a part of the problem as any choice you have made. Compromise involves a choice of change from both sides.

Know and recognize that life is a series of choices. Become aware of all the choices you make each day that either move you forward in life, keep you where you are or even help you to move back a step so that you can see the broader picture. Make choices for yourself that make a difference.

ALLOW OTHERS TO HAVE PROBLEMS

Growth comes from being able to solve and work through challenges and problems. You are given more opportunities than you usually know what to do with every day you stay alive. Life is not selective in seeking you out. Life is willing to offer chances of growth to everyone it touches, not just you. Life allows others to have problems and so should you. Don't try to solve everyone's problems. Allow them to grow through making their own choices, their own mistakes and finding their own successes.

Sometimes as a mother or father you forget how you learned and try to solve your children's problems or be the solution yourself. In doing so you hinder you as well as the other person. If you are focused on what you need to do to solve their problem you are not focused on solving your own challenges or meeting your own opportunities for success and growth. You want to be a good parent, but you need to remind yourself parenting involves teaching. You need, as a parent or a friend to teach more and rescue less. You may know the right answer for you but, at best, you can only guess at the right answer for someone else. You do not know the lessons they need to learn. What they learn may not be the same lesson you had to learn.

A part of this is to "Let the Consequence Follow." When you do things or make a choice you end up with logical or natural consequence, either good or bad. These results help you decide what you like or don't like. The consequences you experience from previous choices influence greatly your next choices. If you liked the consequences you will likely make the same choice again. If you did not like the consequences you probably make a different choice the next time. Too often you may try to stop the consequence of choices from touching the lives of those you love and care about. You might step in to keep the consequence from happening or offer to be the safety net just to make it easier for someone else. You trust yourself to handle the circumstances because you have done it before but you often fear your loved ones are not ready to handle the consequence unless it is favorable. Learn tough love and let the consequence follow. Be there to offer support, if possible, when the other person needs it, but let it happen. Stand back from the situation and look at it from a distance and then allow the events to proceed as they will.

Tough love is just what it says. It is loving the other person enough to allow them to live their life by experiencing consequences and feelings. It is indeed tough to watch others suffer or go through trials without rescuing them. It is tough to teach by example when you know what you do may result in pain or sorrow for them. Tough love is having enough love to allow the other person to have problems, to learn and to grow the same way you have by trial and error. Tough love is letting go and allowing life to happen for someone else and being tough enough to be a spectator as it happens.

STAND BACK AND STEP AWAY

Sometimes you are so close to a situation or another person you cannot see clearly. You need to step back and look form a different perspective, from a distance to fully understand. When you are full of feeling and reacting from emotion first in everything you do, it is time to put emotion aside and step back. Analyze, look at or study what it is you are really feeling and why. Often what you are angry about is not the real problem. You are not angry with the person as much as you may be angry at an action or what is happening is something you thought was over but now is popping up again or simply frustration with yourself. Step back, study and remember past lessons. Is the person you are dealing with acting from the same level of maturity you are expecting?

Standing back and looking at the situation or person that has you stuck or upset allows you breathing room. It is a way of taking a deep breath before going on. Standing back allows you to look at the situation or person from the perspective of someone not caught up in the action. Are the other person's demands or requests realistic? Are they mature, thoughtful, respective requests or at the bottom line are they just the actions of and demands of a little child stamping his foot and throwing a temper tantrum. Just recognizing it from a distance gives you strength to either deal with it differently or to let it go as something that is not able to be worked out at this time or not worth the effort and cost to you. It is imperative you sometimes stand back and look at the situations you are in from the perspective of someone outside the circle of conflict in order to truly understand.

Stepping away is deciding to react or to act from a distance where you can see more clearly. Stepping away may mean giving the problem time to be resolved without your intervention. Stepping away may mean walking away for a time then choosing a better time to face the challenge or create a solution. Stepping away may be the choice to allow someone else to experience pain or joy. Stepping away is a way of being more selective in how, when, where and what problems you choose to participate in at this time.

LET GO AND LET...

Let go and let good in. Let go and let another assist you, reach out to you, or take the burden from you. Let go of the apron strings that bind. Let go of the control, the hate, the anger or whatever it is that is holding you down. Let go of simply being stuck where you are. Let go of the fear and let yourself reach for something or someone. A boy stuck in quicksand has to let go of the struggle in order to reach for the branch to pull himself out with. You have to let go of the anger before you can let the feeling of forgiveness in.

Sometimes you have to just let go period. Put the leaf in the stream and let it float away; then look for a new leaf. Maybe you need to let go of the branch in the middle of the raging river and be swept away by the flow to the edge of the waterfall before falling into pool of quiet water at the bottom. The drop may not be nearly as bad as you think. Let go and let the universe work in its perfection. The universe flows all around you. Let go and allow yourself to flow on the river of life. Let go, enjoy the ride and relax.

MANAGE THE FEELING

STOP DROP AND ROLL

Firemen in the schools teach children that when they are on fire they need to stop, drop and roll. This safety procedure is essential in reducing the risk of severe injury or even death. It is just as important that you use this safety idea when dealing with the fires of life and those fires you allow to burn inside. Sometimes in order to put the fire out you need to stop, drop and roll emotionally.

Stop fretting. Stop fighting. Stop ignoring the burning inside. Stop fanning the flames. Stop and look from a distance at the feelings. Stop and breathe.

Drop the feeling. Drop the control. Drop the energy level you are expending. Drop the issue altogether. Drop to your knees in prayer. Drop to the floor and exercise. Drop down and sleep.

Roll with the punches. Roll along with the consequence. Roll with the new emotion. Roll with the freedom of nothing being there. Roll with the new energy that flows and pushes you on. Roll with laughter. Roll on with life as it goes along. .

Put out the fires in your life according to the firefighters advice. Stop, Drop and Roll.

LIVE THROUGH THE FEELING

It is possible to live through the feeling. It is easy to live through the feelings of joy, excitement and happiness. The energy lifts you up and carries you with it. It is much harder to feel like you can live through the feelings of grief, the pain of abuse or the despair of loneliness. Sometimes when you are in the depths of depression or the self-recrimination of addiction it feels like you can't go on. You may be so discouraged that you don't even want to go on with life. The feeling is so strong you can't feel anything else. I have felt that way before and I am still around to say it is possible to live through the feeling.

Decide to live. Grasp onto life with both hands and hold on tight. Experience the ride through grief with all of its turns from denial, past anger to acceptance. Wrap up in a cozy blanket and live through the tears of rejection or abuse. Scream your way through feelings of frustration and hate. Walk your way through a feeling of being valueless. Read your way through feeling overwhelmed and burdened down. Sign a balloon with all your feelings and let it soar away. Find something you enjoy to help you live through the feelings you don't think you can.

Make friends with the feelings. Recognize any feeling or emotion you have as a part of you. Let your feelings and emotions see the light of day. Don't bury them under a façade of a smile or mask of appropriateness. A buried feeling frequently reappears later as an illness or disability. Acknowledge and love every feeling and emotion you experience. By acknowledging the feelings as they come you can more quickly move from one feeling to another in understanding. For example, you feel angry with a son-in-law because he beat your daughter up during a visit. How dare he do that to her in your own home in front of the grandchildren? You realize the anger is really frustration. You are frustrated and angry because you were not able to stop it before it happened. You find the anger is less due to his physical violence than his turning your home, which the grandchildren see as a safe place to be, into just another battlefield. You move from the frustration of not being able to protect those you love to a feeling of revenge. It is not really revenge felt but a desire to teach him a lesson. You are really just an annoyed parent with one child while on the other hand wanting to protect another. You realize the feeling is of powerlessness and failing to teach them better. Like peeling an onion you go through the feelings. Now you have dealt with the feelings you can focus on something else. In this instance as you turn attention to your daughter you hear crying. She is not crying because she is hurt or because her children are scared. She is crying because her husband walked out without her and she is afraid he might go to one of their friend's without her. All she wants to do is run after him, tell him she knows he is sorry and wants to go with him. As you watch the anger and frustration completely disappears. Now you can almost see a humor in the situation. You may feel frustrated and angry they return and they are sorry, but for now you can recognize these are just two children playing. He stamps his foot for service. She doesn't obey so he has to beat her up. He claims he didn't mean to hurt her. It was just an accident. She agrees with him and they run off to play together at a friend's as though nothing ever happened. You feel a release of emotion as you watch them driving off together laughing and giggling like school kids. You lived through the moment and have found a bit of laughter on the other side. You can use this laughter to help start again as you go in to comfort the children, trying to restore peace, comfort and stable love to their world. It is possible to live through the feelings and be a survivor.

FORGIVE

Forgive yourself. Show love by forgiving yourself for the perceived wrong decisions, mistakes, missed opportunities or low self-esteem you have lived with. Forgive yourself for choices made and choices not made which affected your life, bringing you to the present moment. You often allow others to make mistakes in their lives and love them anyway. You need to give yourself the same love for the same mistakes. Forgive yourself for not being perfect. Forgive yourself for not being the neighbor you idolize or the image you see on TV. What you see is not always reality, but merely what others want you to see. Give yourself love and praise for the good choices you have made and the place you are at today.

Forgive others for perceived hurts, wrongs and mistakes made. Clear your heart and mind to see them as just another human being who made a choice you do not agree with. Forgive them and thank them for acting as a teacher in your life. Forgive without expectation of an apology from them, because in most instances you will not get one. In some situations you may never even have the opportunity to talk to the person you forgive. You must forgive them in your heart for your own personal good and peace. The person you are hurting the most by holding in the feelings of hurt and bitterness is yourself. Love yourself enough to forgive others.

Forgiving is different from forgetting. Forgiving is not making everything all better. You can remember an experience and learn from it, looking back at it often for the lessons of importance in the present while forgiving the person involved you felt hurt or wronged by. Forgiving another means freeing yourself to use the energy you have sustained in hate, anger, hurt or fear toward seeking new goals, reaching for a new image or enjoying life with your family. Forgiving is the act of reaching out in love to someone else with no expectations in return. It is setting the incident of hurt and opening the pathway for a different kind of relationship. The new relationship does not have to be as it once was. That may not be possible. Sometimes the act of forgiveness is just making it possible for you to be in the same room without wanting to run away or wanting to either cry or scream. Think about who you can forgive and find a way to make peace with yourself.

SOMETHING FOR YOU

TREAT YOURSELF

It is important to make time for yourself as well as for others. Treat yourself to something important to you at least once a week. It could be a hot fragrant bubble bath, 15 minutes of uninterrupted reading, watching your favorite movie or sports team or listening to music you enjoy. Perhaps you like to walk alone in the park, dance to an old tune, get a makeover at a local store or simply find a few moments to just put your feet up and meditate in silence or nap. Go for a drive in the country or a picnic at the park. Take yourself to dinner and the theatre without guilt. Whatever makes you feel special, allow it to happen. Schedule time for yourself, then keep the appointment.

STOP AND BE A CHILD

Be a Child. Let the child out to play, to explore to learn anew. It is easy to get busy with life and duties and roles you think are important and forget that life doesn't have to be so rushed, hurried and scheduled. When the child at your knee asks you to look at something, take a moment or more to look though the eyes of a child. Let yourself become a child and see the wonderment of life as you did when you were younger. Look at the picture without judgment or learned beliefs. Sit down and draw a picture from a child's perspective of newness and freedom of will where any color is okay and expression is the center of life and exciting. Take a moment while watering the plant to see the flower as a miracle springing from the earth for the sheer joy of just being pretty. Be a child and count the petals on a daisy or the colors on a butterfly's wing. Throw, kick or catch a ball with abandonment.

Being a child is being free. It is seeing more before you and hope for nothing but good. Allow yourself to feel this hope, newness and open perspective regularly. You can't be a happy child and a stressed out adult at the same time. Relieve the stress by choosing into allowing the child freedom to heal and to live. A child doesn't hold grudges for long periods of time. A child easily forgives and desires forgiveness of others. A child is free enough to be able to say "I'm sorry" without worrying about how it looks to someone else. Most children do not regularly hurt others just to get power. They reach out to others. A child values the freedom of having many friends to choose from and returns the friendship innocently, without expectation. A child allows himself freedom to learn and to play in the same day.

A child believes that life was made for him to enjoy, so he looks for ways to enjoy life. He looks for ways to make his world better. He looks for life to bring him the things that he needs or wants and waits for them to simply show up. He expects miracles to come his way. A child is also flexible and changeable. It is perfectly okay to want to be a fireman one day and a doctor the next. If a dream doesn't come true when expected they simply look for another dream to wish for. Time is of little matter. They don't worry about what they are late for. They want to know how much more time they have for enjoying amusement activities. You need to look at your world through the expectant eyes of a child. Look with wonder and belief that anything is possible.

LAUGH AT LIFE

Don't be afraid to find the humor in the situation or the feeling. Sometimes the humor is easy to find, it hits you right in the forehead and tickles all the way down. More often than not you need to look for the humor.

Laugh at yourself. Admit when you do something unexpected or outrageous and laugh. Laugh at a choice you just can't believe you made. Find the humor in the simple things that happen to you. Start your day with a smile. Look in the mirror at your hair first thing in the morning. Have you seen anything funnier on a clown in a parade or the circus? Have you ever stumbled through the house in the dark so you wouldn't wake anyone by turning on the light? Laugh at the number of things you bumped into or knocked over on your little adventure. Laugh at your own reactions to others. Can you laugh at the embarrassing moment at work or the comment to your friend that didn't sound at all the way you meant it? There is probably at least one incident each day that you could find to laugh at.

Like stepping back, looking for the humor allows you to change your feeling. Look beneath what is in front of you and find something to relieve the pain. Is your daughter throwing a temper tantrum you are having a hard time dealing with? Then look at the cute or funny faces she is making and inwardly let yourself laugh and enjoy the moment. Does your son take clean clothes and put them back into the laundry to avoid putting them away? You can either get irritated about it or laugh at the weekly game you play together. When your grandchild spilled the milk while getting his own drink did you choose to feel overwhelmed because of the mess or could you see the humor in his standing there with milk dripping over the glass and down his arm? When faced with two possible feelings, choose laughter. It lasts longer and lightens the spirit.

KEEP THE SCALES IN BALANCE

Life is full of opposites: good and bad, happy and sad, boring and exciting. It is okay to experience it all. You should experience it all as you travel through life. When you look around at the workings of nature marvel at the balance of life. Winter snows are the balance to summer heat. We too can achieve balance in our lives.

Create balance between work and play. It is said, with truth, "All Work and No Play Makes Jack a Dull Boy." If the scales are tipping down because work is pressuring you and duties overwhelm, then balance the scales by seeking out the laughter of a good joke, the splash of a puddle, the smile of a friend. If you work for eight hours at a stress filled job, make the rest of your day as stress free as possible. Listen to a story on tape or your favorite music during your commutes. Sing a song as you prepare your meals. Listen to a child read and enjoy the escape to a fantasy world.

Scales are very much like a teeter-totter as children play. Sometimes you are up, sometimes you are down and sometimes you are in perfect balance. It takes effort but the excitement far outweighs the cost. When you are down you have to work, push up, to find the balance. You might be on the down side, feeling the grief and sorrow of separation. In order to get back up you push. You visit a widow down the street, sharing with her compassion and understanding of her loneliness. Together you come into balance for a short while. As you leaves, she shares with you how much your visit meant to her. Without doing anything more than receiving her gift you go higher until you are all the way up. Now it is life's turn to push. As life pushes back and you descend think about the fun you are having. Enjoy the ride down as much as you did the ride up. Decide how far down you want to go. You can go all the way down until you hit the bottom with a thud or push back up as soon as your feet touch the ground. How you play the game is up to you. You decide how or when to balance the ride.

Keep the scales in balance emotionally and physically. Waking and sleeping are opposites of your day. Take as much care to enjoy your sleep as you do your day. Exercise and playing with the family is your counter to long hours at a desk. Sometimes you can even experience the opposites together. As you mow the lawn (the work) take time to look around at nature and enjoy the chance to walk through your yard, smell the flowers and get a little exercise (the fun).. While you are washing the dishes don't forget to play with the fresh bubbles. Find your own personal ways of balancing the emotions of your days. Counter each down with an up and stay in balance. Balance hurt and discouragement out by giving love and encouragement to yourself or someone else.

FILL THE TANKS OFTEN

You can only give away what you have to give. You can only run if you have the energy to run on. A well running automobile is dependent on fuel in the tank, oil in the engine and a fully charged battery. Just like the car, you have within holding tanks you draw from to run well and smoothly. You cannot give love if you do not have love inside. You cannot strengthen others if you have no strength of your own left. You cannot give service if you have not received service from others.

Identify your tanks. Ask yourself, what is it I give away? What are the ways I support others? What do I teach others is important in life? As you answer these questions you will find the tanks of love you draw from. Some of my personal tanks are: Love for self, Love for others, Patience, Service, Faith & Hope, Strength and Belief.

The ways to fill the tank are simple. The biggest way is to find ways to love yourself, Do things for you that build self-esteem, patience, strength and calm. Seek out those who touch you. Allow their energy, their enthusiasm, their service or their encouragement to energize you, to fill you up and renew you. Seek out books, movies and music that inspire, enrich or you simply enjoy.

You can't overfill the tanks. You can only share the extra. As you learn to fill your tanks you will find you have more and more to give away. It becomes an act of recycling. You receive a hug from your daughter and pass it on to your son. You receive inspiration from a book you read and share it with a friend. You feel free to give away any part of your reserve because you know you can refill it with ease as often as necessary.

SERVE SOMEONE ELSE

Lose yourself in thoughts of someone else. There is always someone else who needs a helping hand, a word of encouragement or could benefit from an act of kindness. You are not alone in your loneliness, your despair, your frustrations or your trials. I learned many years ago that no matter what I thought I could not live through much longer, there was always someone who was living with something worse. I might be dealing with sexual abuse but I hadn't been physically scarred by it yet. I might have three children with a hereditary bone disease but at least they had the hope of walking normally for a part of their lives. Thinking of these other women, I was able to find ways to reach out to them and let them know they were not alone. In reaching out I forgot my own pain. My burdens seemed more bearable. My focus turned outward rather than inward and healing began.

Sometimes just looking for someone else to touch and to reach out to is all you need in order to know deep within that you have something left. When you feel there is nothing else you can give to yourself or to anyone else in your life, the desire to give to someone else is sometimes the catalyst that allows you to realize there is more within that has not been tapped into. Giving away a piece of love, a smile or a pat on the back for someone else, allows you to reach into that inner reservoir and uncap the hidden treasures. Once found, you and others can use those treasures to heal and strengthen each other.

BE GRATEFUL

There is always something to be grateful for. No matter what our circumstances, we can find something good about it. Long ago I was admonished to "Be grateful for small favors, however small they may be." I use this piece of advice almost everyday. In finding something small to be thankful for, I am able to change my energy from negative to positive in a fraction of a second. It has never failed to lift my spirits and allow me to see my circumstances and trials from a better perspective.

Look for the things to be grateful for in the very circumstances that are burdening you down. You may not have much more than a loaf of bread and a jar of peanut butter to feed the children, but you can be grateful to the person who donated it to the food kitchen. You may not have a steady job but you have extra time to be with your family. Be thankful for simply being alive. Be thankful for waking up each morning, no matter where you are, to a new day. Be thankful for being able to walk, see, hear, speak and breathe with ease. Look for the little things in life each day. Look around you, at yourself and those you love. Find something everyday to be thankful for. .

It is often the hardest times of our lives that we get to be thankful for. When my children were young, I got to spend many hours in the hospital with some of them following surgeries. The hours were long and the children got bored easily. During this time I was grateful to find that I had an ability to make up stories to share with them and their roommates to fill the hours with happiness. I was grateful for being able to create and teach other mothers learning games and activities constructed from the very medical supplies that some of the children feared. Although these years brought many challenges they also were some of my most creative periods. My son does not remember much of what those years were like, but the nurses that cared for him still remember the stories and games I created when he would respond to no one else. I was not wise enough to make multiple copies of the stories I gave away so I would have them to share again but I am grateful knowing they touched other families for unknown periods throughout the years.

WRITE IT DOWN

Write it down and work it through. Writing is one of best therapies I have ever found. When you do not know what it is that is bothering you, simply find a piece of paper and a pencil and start writing. Write whatever comes to your mind. Don't judge the thoughts. Just write them down. You will be surprised how quickly the words come as you give yourself permission to allow the thoughts to flow randomly and unchecked. Don't worry whether the thoughts are positive or negative. Don't worry whether they even make sense. Just write. When your mind begins to slow or the words stop coming then stop. Pause. Now read what you have written. You will find as you write you discover what the issue is burdening or worrying you. You will find you have many feelings about what to do and how to feel. Generally by the time you have finished writing you will even have found a workable solution to a problem or at the least, the first steps to take.

Write it down and remember. It doesn't matter whether it is a scrapbook, a notebook or a journal. Find someway to help you remember the good times. Remembering the times of success, joy and happiness assure you can find your way through the trial and past the obstacle presently in your life. Write down the special hug your son gave you as he ran in from school. Write down the time you laughed at yourself as you arrived at church and found you had put on one black shoe and one dark blue shoe and didn't have time to go home and change before playing the piano during the meeting. Write down the time you said no to helping with the PTA drive and spent the night playing board games with your family. Write down the excitement of making your first pie or finding the perfect cookie recipe. Write down the day you got on the scale and found you had lost two pounds without even trying. Whatever it is that will give you strength, faith and hope at a later time, write it down now so you can remember it later.

IT IS PERFECT

This moment is here as it is. You have created the past and can achieve something different in the future, but right now is the perfect moment that you have created for yourself. Why would you create something for yourself that is less than perfect? Accept that in some way this moment you have created is perfect.

This moment is perfect. Where you are in life at this moment is perfect. Whatever you are doing at this moment is perfect. Whatever challenges are being faced at the moment are perfect for you. Whatever joy and happiness are in your life at this moment is perfect. The people in your life at this moment are perfectly in place. This moment is perfect in every way. At this moment you are the perfect weight, in the perfect place to be, doing exactly what you should be doing.

Open yourself up to the belief that every moment is perfect in some way. It may not always feel or look perfect by the standards you use, but it is perfect in some way. Every moment is perfect for someone that is there. Even when a moment is filled with fear or ill feelings it is perfect because someone is learning a lesson, making a choice or changing as a result. Even feeling threatened or abused may be the perfect moment that gives you the strength or reason to change circumstances you no longer want. Have you ever been in line at a grocery store when a person in front of you does not have the exact change he needs for his purchases? To the person without the money the moment may not seem perfect. However the moment is perfect for one person to touch the life of another. Every person behind him has the perfect opportunity to reach out in love and offer a penny or two to assist.

Accept who you are, what you are, where you are, how you are and why you are at this moment as perfect for some reason you may have yet to learn about.

BUILD A BRIDGE FOR OTHERS

Look behind you at the steps you have taken as you made this journey. Perhaps as you crossed the boards they creaked with age. One or two may have felt a little wobbly and you wondered whether to trust them or not. Was there one you were not sure would hold up under the weight of your problems or circumstances? Did you find the board that appeared new to you? Did you notice the new board surrounded by ones weathered by the elements as during times they served others passing over? Which one did you recognize as a skill you admire in someone you respect or wish you were more like? Which one did you almost skip or step over thinking you didn't need it but decided to give it a try anyway because you might miss something? As with any bridge it is not one board alone that gets you from one place to another but side by side they work to make your passage possible and easier than you imagined. As you crossed from one side to another you even enjoyed the journey.

Now it is your turn. You have made it to here to here. Take anything you can and build a bridge for someone else. Pass on a smile, a compliment or a hug. Be an example to others. Inspire someone to follow you in growth and change. Share and teach someone you know something you learned here or through experience.

Be a Bridge Builder.

Contact:
Linda Chatelain
6289 So. Balsa Circle
West Jordan, UT 84081

Version 2
Published September 2013

www.ingramcontent.com/pod-product-compliance
Lightning Source LLC
Chambersburg PA
CBHW060652030426

42337CB00017B/2570